Make the Pool Your Gym

Make the Pool Your Gym

*No-Impact Water Workouts for Getting Fit,
Building Strength and Rehabbing from Injury*

DR. KARL KNOPF

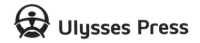

Published in the United States by
Ulysses Press
P.O. Box 3440
Berkeley, CA 94703
www.ulyssespress.com

ISBN: 978-1-61243-014-0
Library of Congress Control Number 2011934782

Printed in the United States by United Graphics Inc.
10 9 8 7 6

Acquisitions: Kelly Reed
Managing editor: Claire Chun
Editor: Lily Chou
Proofreader: Lauren Harrison
Indexer: Sayre Van Young
Production: Judith Metzener
Cover design: what!design @ whatweb.com
Photographs: © Alan Chun except on page 12 © marema/shutterstock.com
Models: Kitty Chiu, Chris Knopf, Karl Knopf, Sasha Wozniak

Distributed by Publishers Group West

Please Note
This book has been written and published strictly for informational purposes, and in no way should be used as a substitute for actual instruction with qualified professionals. The author and publisher are providing you with information in this work so that you can have the knowledge and can choose, at your own risk, to act on that knowledge. The author and publisher also urge all readers to be aware of their health status and to consult health care professionals before beginning any health program.

table of contents

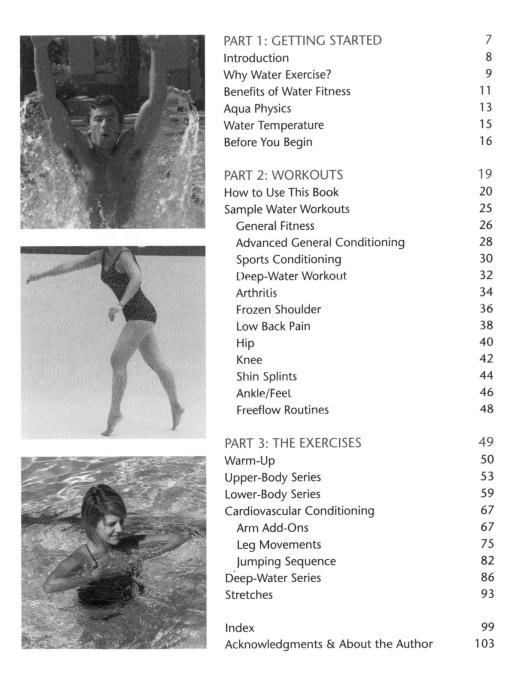

getting
started

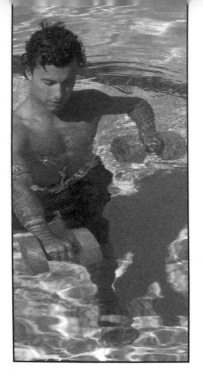

introduction

Water is a critical component of life. Yet when most people hear the word "water," they think of hydration. In *Make the Pool Your Gym*, we show you how to exercise in it—beyond the old standby of swimming. The ability to swim is not required, and you don't even need to get your hair wet. Water workouts are a sensible and comprehensive way to exercise without subjecting the body to the same stress that's placed on it during land-based programs.

The beauty of water exercise is that it can accommodate the fitness needs of everyone. It's generally considered safe for people with arthritis and musculoskeletal problems, and warm water is very beneficial for people with joint stiffness and pain.

Water exercise is not just land exercise in the water. However, just like land-based exercise programs, water fitness benefits range from helping to control blood sugar levels to improving aerobic fitness. A study in 2009 found that aquatic exercise helped relieve chronic back pain more effectively than land programs. Water exercise has also been proven to be helpful for pregnant women with back pain.

Whether you're a serious athlete, a fitness enthusiast, a beginner, or someone with a chronic condition, water exercise can efficiently improve cardiovascular performance and strength in a very short amount of time. It's ideal for cross-training or a total-body workout, and can also be used as an introductory mode of exercise.

Make the Pool Your Gym invites you to explore this safe and effective alternative way to get—and stay—fit. If you're tired of workouts that leave you feeling more battered than better, water workouts may be the solution.

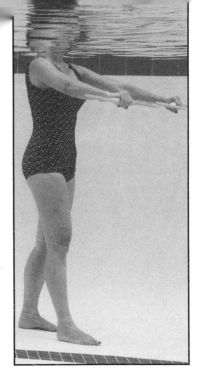

why water exercise?

Water exercise isn't new; it's been around since 200 B.C. Much of the current field of aquatic rehabilitation has its roots in the European and early American spa world. Social bathing was also an important part of ancient Greek and Roman culture. Since earliest recorded history, water has been believed to promote healing and has been widely used in the management of medical ailments.

Natural springs and water therapies became a central focus of many health spas and healers from all backgrounds, who noted the positive effects of water on various medical conditions. It's through observation and centuries of trial and error that today's scientific methodology of aquatic treatments have evolved.

The popularity of water classes has increased from 500,000 in the 1990s to over 4 million today, with the water fitness movement partly fueled by the aquatic rehabilitation exercises done by high-profile athletes such as Nancy Kerrigan, Bo Jackson and Carl Lewis. The beauty of a water workout is that it serves both ends of the fitness spectrum, from people with severe chronic conditions to world-class athletes. Note that you don't need to be a swimmer to do water workouts—non-swimmers or people who don't want to get their hair wet can take aquatic classes in shallow, waist-deep water.

Water fitness has a long list of benefits and a very short one of risks, and current wellness educators are looking at the aquatic environment as a safe, effective and inexpensive way to preserve health and treat disease. It's the "open door" to health and wellness for many people who have limited abilities and chronic conditions. In addition to its role in rehabilitation and physical therapy, water exercise can also provide a strenuous workout for elite athletes.

Advantages of Water Fitness over Land Exercise

Water workouts offer numerous advantages over land workouts. Some high-level trainers use water as a method to engage in

WATER EXERCISE VS. SWIMMING

While swimming is an excellent vehicle for building muscle tone and endurance, it's limited to using the same set of muscles over and over again. Water exercise offers far more options and goes from horizontal to vertical, thus providing a comprehensive workout in multiple planes. This means participants can perform motions in any and all angles not available on standard exercise machines. The goal of any well-rounded workout is to provide a total-body workout that engages major muscle group. Because water provides natural resistance to body movements, water exercises strengthen complementary muscle groups simultaneously. No land-based routine is as time efficient.

sports conditioning or as a way to employ plyometrics. Since water is far denser than air, water can apply up to 12 times greater resistance. The harder you push and pull during a water workout, the more productive it becomes. The resistance of water challenges beginners to highly conditioned athletes alike. Fortunately, water workouts have a built-in safety feature that land workouts lack. Since the amount of resistance in water depends on the speed of movement, you can't create more resistance than your body can tolerate.

Heart rates during water exercise are lower than during land-based training but you can still obtain the same physiological benefits with less heart-pounding exercise. Despite this, the common belief that water workouts burn less fat and fewer calories than other exercise is false. Aquatic aerobics can burn 400 to 700 calories an hour—about the same as land-based aerobics, but all without placing any strain on the joints while stimulating circulation. One recent study found that a one-hour water exercise session performed at a moderate pace expends the same amount of calories as walking for one hour at a pace of 3 miles per hour.

A Kinder, Gentler Way to Fitness

A decade ago, aqua exercise classes were few and far between and, when people heard the term "water exercise," they thought of ladies at the retirement home doing simple moves. Today, water exercise is no longer just for grandmas. While water is the perfect element for people with joint problems to exercise in because it diminishes the effects of gravity and allows movements that would be painful and difficult on land to be performed with greater ease, it offers several advantages over land, including greater buoyancy and better resistance, plus being a whole lot more enjoyable.

Standing in neck-deep water, a person weighs about 10 percent of what he or she does on land. This effect, coupled with the cushioning property of water, places less pressure on the joints. This is especially beneficial to arthritis sufferers, athletes with joint or overuse injuries, and overweight people. Weekend warriors who are beat up from overtraining but won't take a day off for fear of de-conditioning might consider cross-training in water to maintain their fitness level. Some athletes can improve performance by taking time off to cross-train in the pool. Non-impact deep-water running, for instance, has been proven to successfully hasten cardiovascular performance in athletes with overuse injuries.

Please note, however, that while water exercise is good for most people, there are some conditions under which water workouts should not be performed:

- severe hypertension or hypotension
- cardiac conditions
- infectious skin disorders

It's always wise to consult your health care professional for your specific recommendations.

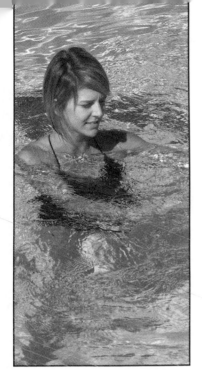

benefits of water fitness

Recent research has shown that many of the health conditions seen today can be positively influenced by regular exercise and proper nutrition. This is where water fitness enters the scene. Not only can it be performed by most of the population, it provides social and psychological benefits as well as physiological ones.

Some of the health issues that can be improved through water exercise include musculoskeletal problems (low back pain, spinal compression, bone loss), neurological problems (e.g., Parkinson's disease, multiple sclerosis), cardiopulmonary pathology (emphysema) and ambulatory conditions (e.g., severe arthritis of the hip or knee, peripheral artery disease).

Physiological Benefits
- Improved muscular strength and endurance
- Increased functional flexibility

- Expanded cardiovascular fitness
- Decreased pain
- Decreased impact on joints
- Decreased risk of injury
- Improved sleep patterns
- Hastened recovery time from injuries
- Better posture and body mechanics
- Reduced risk for chronic diseases

Social and Psychological Benefits
- Improved self-efficacy and self-esteem
- Reduced pain on expanded movements

- Increased social interaction and new friendships
- Opportunity to develop social support
- Reduced tension and stress
- Improved sleep
- Decreased fatigue

A well-designed water exercise program works both agonist and antagonist muscle groups (e.g., biceps brachii/triceps brachii, hamstrings/quadriceps) with just one simple exercise, which means you can work out your whole body in half the time—perfect for people with busy schedules. Water exercise is isokinetic,

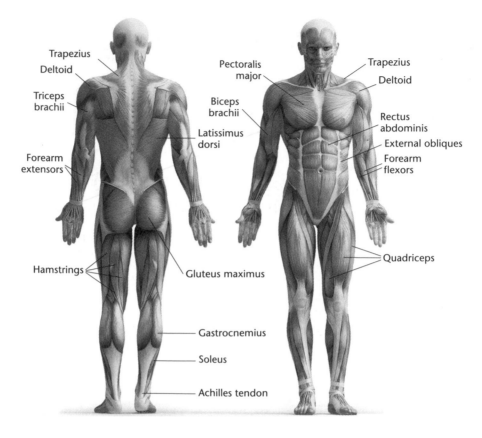

Trapezius
Deltoid
Triceps brachii
Forearm extensors
Hamstrings
Gluteus maximus
Gastrocnemius
Soleus
Achilles tendon

Pectoralis major
Biceps brachii
Latissimus dorsi
Trapezius
Deltoid
Rectus abdominis
External obliques
Forearm flexors
Quadriceps

Major Muscles

which means that the resistance stays consistent through full range of motion. In addition, it allows you to perform multi-directional moves that are more practical but not possible on weight machines.

No special equipment is needed to get a tremendous workout. Deep-water options such as aqua jogging can really challenge the cardiovascular system of even highly motivated people. To adjust load and resistance in exercises, simply change the angle of your arms or hands and alter the speed of the movement. If you want to further intensify the work, you can wear aqua gloves or use variable resistance-training devices (VRTDs).

After years of designing and implementing therapeutic exercise programs, I'm convinced that the social aspects of a water fitness class are just as enriching and satisfying as the physiological improvements. The walk-away feeling that you had fun and felt good while doing something that's positive for your health and fitness is what makes water exercisers continue to participate, rain or shine.

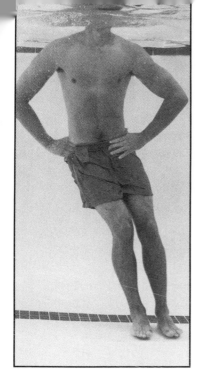

aqua physics

To successfully engage in a water exercise program, you don't need to be an expert in hydrodynamics, but understanding the basics of how water can influence your work is helpful. The secret to being an effective water fitness participant is to know how and when to employ the correct concepts and tools to elicit the correct outcome. The key to designing an effective water routine is to adapt the physical properties of water principles to meet your personal fitness needs.

Too many land exercisers think that water exercise is just land exercises done in the pool. However, the forces applied in the water are very different than on land. As an example, clap your hands quickly together and spread them apart on land, then do that same move in the water. You'll see how, when performed in the water, resistance is applied throughout the full range of motion in both directions.

There are a number of principles, such as drag, buoyancy, density and water temperature, that will impact your work in the water. We'll just briefly tackle a few of them.

Buoyancy gives water exercise its "soft" capacity, which reduces compression and weight bearing on joints. The depth of the water influences the compression placed upon the body: the deeper you stand in the water, the more buoyancy plays a role in lifting you off the floor of the pool. For instance, if you stand in neck-deep water, you'll weigh only 10% of your body weight; if you stand in waist-deep water, you'll weigh 50% of your body weight. Thus the deeper you go, the less you weigh.

Water's *resistance* allows exercises to be easily and gradually adjusted based on speed, levers and surface area. Using a bigger variable resistance-training device (VRTD) or simply opening your hand increases resistance; however, slicing your open hand through the water creates less-intense movement than either a fist or an open hand that impacts the water with the palm.

Resistance exerted on the surface straight on is called "frontal tension." Because of frontal tension, you can more easily walk sideways than straight ahead in the water, and more easily slice your hand through the water than slap it. You can increase frontal resistance by either moving more quickly

14

forward/backward, or placing a kickboard sideways then running forward.

When performing exercise on land, "gravity" is the primary force we must overcome. When in the water, *drag* is the resistance you encounter as you move through it. Drag is the primary force that governs our approach in the water. The density of the water coupled with drag creates greater resistance for the exerciser. The faster you move in the water, the more drag you create. For aquatic exercise, drag and turbulence are beneficial tools for increasing resistance and building strength. Drag shielding is also known as "drafting," an effect seen when there's a line of one or more people or objects in the water or on land. Drafting decreases the frontal resistance/intensity for all but the first person. This concept is useful when performing rehabilitation such as gait training.

The following compares the significant factors that influence land exercise and water exercise:

On Land	In the Water
Gravity	Drag
Acceleration	Buoyancy
Impact	Hydrostatic pressure

The more abruptly you move through water, the more *turbulence* you'll create. A person who is physically limited may want to limit turbulence as much as possible to limit any additional resistance. An elite runner, on the other hand, may want to create as much turbulence as possible to increase resistance, which is not possible on land.

Motion occurs when there's a change of location in space, and can be linear (right to left, forward to back, etc.) or rotational (flexion, extension, adduction, abduction). With water exercise, you can apply resistance in any direction that's physically possible. Acceleration (the rate of change of velocity/speed) is one component of motion. It'll require more effort/power for you to apply a new sudden burst of movement than just continuing a movement at the same pace. This approach can be applied as a conditioning tool (for example, quickly running forward five feet, stopping and reversing directions can be a challenging workout).

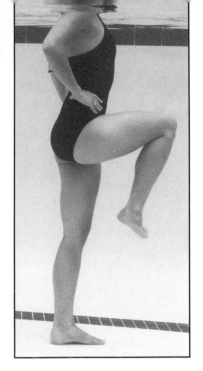

water temperature

Everyone has a preference when it comes to water temperature. A person with arthritis or joint pain will prefer warm water, a client with MS might prefer cooler water, while a person who wants a vigorous workout will tolerate a cooler water temperature. Understanding the effects of water temperatures will increase your compliance rates and enjoyment.

When the lifeguard stands on the deck and says, "Don't complain, the water's fine. It's 80 degrees," clearly she doesn't understand water temperature. Water facilitates the transfer of heat or cold more quickly than air, which means a water temperature of 75°F will seem much colder than an air temperature of 75°F. Most experts agree that skin temperature is approximately 93°F and anything less than that is going to feel cooler to your skin. This is why some people take a cold shower before jumping in the pool, while others may opt to wear a lightweight wet suit.

The most comfortable temperature range for water aerobics is 80 to 84°F. If the pool is cooler than this, you'll need to warm up for a longer time and will probably want to conduct your flexibility exercises following the aerobic phase instead of at the end of workout. Pool temperatures warmer than 86 to 88°F can be hazardous for vigorous workouts.

Each type of workout has an ideal water temperature:
- Arthritis/therapy classes: 83–88°F
- Competitive athletic classes: 80–83°F
- Stretch and relax classes: 83–86°F

Most multi-purpose pools are kept at 82°F. Keep in mind that swimmers generally like the pool cooler and, with the cost of energy getting higher, the pool manager is not likely to increase the temperature to your ideal range. Therefore, the best suggestion is to adapt your workout rather than fight to get the pool temperature to ideal levels. If exercising in an outdoor pool in cool weather, consider wearing a hat or even a lightweight, short wet suit.

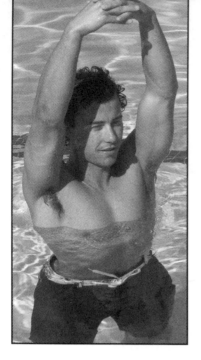

before you begin

Before you start a water-fitness program, it's critical that you're water safe. Even though you don't need to be a swimmer, you need to be able to keep yourself above water and swim/paddle to a safe area if you lose your footing. Entry into the pool will almost always feel cool, so a shower beforehand or a light wet suit can make the transition easier. Once in the pool, most people feel so good they often overdo it. Start out very slowly and progress from a safe foundation.

Water exercise heart rates don't need to be as high as land-based exercise heart rates, so keep that in mind while you work out. The "talk test" is the best approach to follow when doing water exercise—if you can't talk while exercising, you're working too hard, but if you can debate a hot topic, you're not working hard enough. As always, consult your health professional for any specific guidelines for your health condition.

Safety

While none of the exercises in this book will absolutely hurt every person, research has shown that over time, chronic use of any movement can exacerbate an orthopedic condition. In addition, although water exercise is generally safe for everyone, a few conditions (infectious skin disorders, severe high/low blood pressure, some heart issues) may be precluded from an aquatic fitness environment. It's always wise when in doubt to consult a physician before performing water workouts.

Let's review certain protocols that should be taken to have a great, safe workout. Always make sure your body is ready for movement with an adequate warm-up. Do your best to maintain proper posture when performing any water exercise. Listen to your body and never overdo it. If exercising outdoors, stay alert to air quality and pollution, and make sure you protect your skin.

Remember to breathe normally during exercise—don't hold your breath, which is something many people unknowingly do when doing the strength portion of a water exercise class. Counting, talking or singing along with the movement encourages breathing.

Some water aerobics classes use music in their program. Consider standing away the speakers to preserve your hearing and to actually hear the instructor's commands.

When you're done with your workout, continue with low-intensity exercise (such as water walking) to encourage the proper return of blood to your heart. This will prevent any "pooling" effect that may occur in the lower extremities. Never leave the pool with a high, exercise-induced heart rate and *never* jump into the sauna or hot tub while you have a high exercise heart rate or elevated blood pressure.

Exercises to Be Careful With

Even if you think you're in great physical shape, you should still pay attention to your body when performing water workouts. All it takes is one wrong movement to give yourself a chronic condition. Possible high-risk areas include the shoulders, low back, hips and knees.

Arms/Shoulders

- Straighten arms slowly and smoothly—avoid hyper-

Many professional and world-class athletes use water to maintain their fitness when injured. Some factors to keep in mind when using water to rehabilitate a sports injury:

- Follow the advice of a physician and/or therapist.
- Exercise unaffected areas until you're approved for exercising injured areas.
- Cross-train—exercise both agonist and antagonist muscle groups.
- Develop your workout to exercise muscles that replicate the specific sport requirements and movements.
- If painful, slow down the movement and decrease the range of motion.
- Make increases in resistance and speed slowly.
- Use visualization, variations and fun to keep workouts enjoyable and challenging.

extending or hyperflexing the elbow joint (this means no snapping the arms straight).
- Keep your hands where you can see them. Any time your hands are out of sight, you're at potential risk of causing trauma to the shoulder joint.
- Avoid adding resistance equipment before you're ready.

Low back

- Regardless of the movement you perform, you should always maintain good neutral spine posture.
- Perform straight-leg swings slowly and with control to prevent your spine from twisting; keep your abs tight.
- When doing flutter kicks while holding onto a kickboard or the edge of the pool, keep your back, neck and shoulders protected.

Some people find using a snorkel helpful in preventing the low back arch.

Hips

- Perform straight-leg extensions slowly and smoothly, and only raise the leg to hip height.
- Bringing your knees higher than hip height or 90° may cause issues if you have hip problems or osteoporosis.

Knees

- Avoiding using resistance devices on your legs if you have knee issues.
- Keep your knee centered over your ankle and bent no more than 90° when lunging to the side or front.

Equipment

As stated earlier, you don't need any special equipment to reap the benefits of water exercise. Both an open hand and a closed hand

I once had a lady in my class who was 150 pounds overweight and hated exercise. I told her she only had to come to class for 15 minutes and then she could leave if she wanted. Funny thing is, after she was in class for 15 minutes and laughing with the other ladies, I told her to leave. She wouldn't leave and said, "Since I'm wet already, I might as well stay." (Mind you, this was in an outdoor pool in January in California.)

We took the 15-minute concept one step farther. I told her that she could eat anything she wanted *but* she needed to wait 15 minutes. If after 15 minutes she still wanted to eat it, she could. Funny thing is, usually after 15 minutes, she got distracted by something else and didn't still want the thing.

So please remember: The key to better health and wellness is having a realistic goal and being regular. You probably wouldn't neglect brushing your teeth daily so don't neglect your exercise daily!

can generate adequate resistance to give you a good workout. The secret to effective water exercise are the 3 S's: *speed* (the faster you move, the more resistance you generate), *size/surface area* (the larger the surface area of the object, the more resistance), and *shape* of the object.

Popular variable resistance-training devices (VRTDs) include gloves, hard hand paddles and flotation paddles. A solid device, such as plastic paddles with adjustable fins, will generally give you an all–around better workout than something that floats to the top of the pool (e.g., soft foam paddles), thus doing a portion of the work for you. Aqua gloves can be worn throughout an exercise routine and are reasonably priced.

For deep-water exercise, noodles are a good, inexpensive option. Aqua steps are available if you want to do step aerobics. There are even treadmills and stationary bikes built for the pool.

Each prop has advantages and disadvantages. If you choose to use them, you'll quickly find the piece(s) of equipment that work best for you. Most of these items can be purchased online or at sporting goods stores or even pool supply outlets.

part 2
workouts

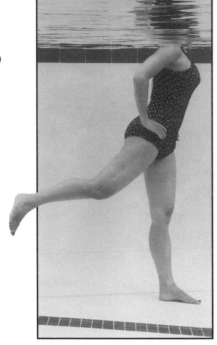

how to use this book

This section of *Make the Pool Your Gym* presents workouts (starting on page 25) for a number of training goals and physical conditions. Pick the one that best suits your needs, or use the samples as springboards for creating your own routine. The sample workouts are designed so that you start with a warm-up and progress to move advanced exercises. All exercise descriptions are provided in Part 3. If you prefer creating your own workout, you can do that too.

Designing a Water-Fitness Workout

The beauty of a water-fitness program is that there really are no rules. No one can see what's going on below the surface so, as long as you feel fine, go for it. Your body and the water will tell you what's best for you. Too often water-fitness instructors make up complicated routines solely for the purpose of keeping themselves from getting bored. Your heart, lungs and muscles don't care if the routine is choreographed or basic. The perfect workout is the one you enjoy while you're doing it, and makes you feel good afterward.

When I do my own routine, I'll mix and match my favorite leg exercises with my favorite arm movements; I switch the combinations depending on how my body responds to the work. Most of us have selected water exercise for a reason, perhaps because our joints hurt, we've overtrained on land, or it's too hot to go out for a run. When it comes to water fitness, enjoy the process—be creative and playful. Train, don't strain!

Fit Tip: If you have a cold, most doctors say it's OK to exercise if the symptoms are above the throat.

While the above may sound fine for some, I know many people want guidelines. Here are some suggestions for designing a fun and fabulous fitness workout.

Start with a Thermal Warm-Up

Begin with a thermal warm-up to increase your core temperature and prepare your muscles for motion. Usually this takes 5–10 minutes and includes water walking in all directions with breaststroke arms. I also call this portion "inventory check-in time." While you walk, check which parts of your body are clicking and which parts are clunking. After the inventory check, you should know which parts of your body need TLC that day. Many people like to spend a few minutes afterward doing some gentle moves/stretches to ready the body for movement. If you feel fine, just progress to the next section of the routine, but make sure you stretch at the end of your routine to foster your flexibility, whether you do so in the pool, the hot tub or on land.

Train with Your Goal in Mind

If your focus is increased range of motion in specific joints, perform the gentle motions that address your needs.

If your focus is aerobic exercise, plan on doing 30–40 minutes of cardiovascular movements. This can be a combination of shallow- and deep-water exercises, or just one type. After your cardio work, spend 1–5 minutes allowing your heart to return to your pre-exercise heart rate. Remember: Aquatic heart rates are about 10–15 beats per minute less than your terrestrial target heart rate. If the weather and pool are warm, you may do some gentle stretches or balance work; otherwise, progress directly to resistance work.

If your goal is to tone and strengthen your body, find a resistance that challenges your muscles so that by 30 seconds,

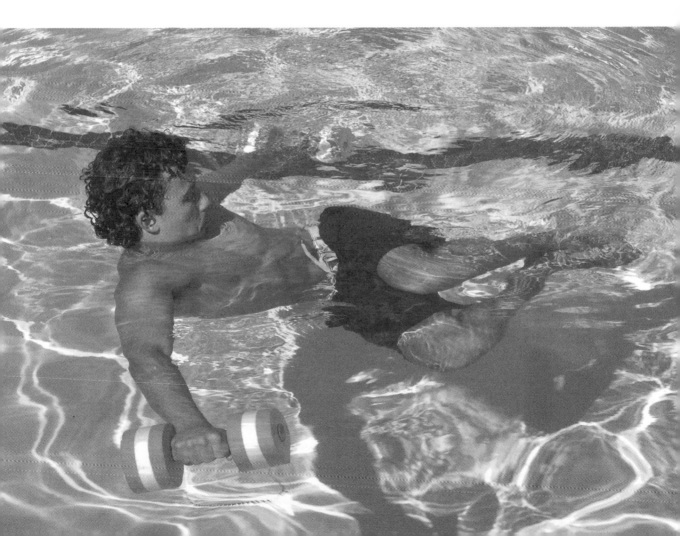

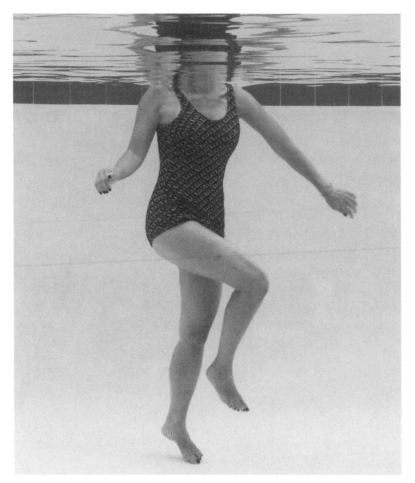

warming up before your workout. A sudden cessation of aerobic activity may cause blood to pool in your lower extremities, which deprives the brain and heart of oxygenated blood and can cause light-headedness or nausea. Thus, it's critical to return your heart rate to pre-exercise levels. To perform your cool-down, walk slowly back and forth in the pool or just swim at a very relaxed pace for about 5 minutes or until your heart rate returns to the pre-exercise level.

Finish with Stretching

Concentrate on the large muscles, such as hamstrings, calves, shoulders and lower back. Stay mindful that when stretching in the pool, you may get chilled, which may prevent you from holding a stretch for as long as is needed. In this case, stretching may need to be done inside a warm place. Here are some stretching tips:

- Perform stretches while standing in shoulder-deep water, breathing slowly and rhythmically in through your nose and out through your mouth.
- To avoid straining ligaments, keep all joints slightly bent/ flexed while moving in a controlled manner and in proper alignment. Protect your spine at all times (i.e., keep your knees relaxed and your pelvis tilted).

your muscles feel like they've been exercised. Eventually work up to doing 3 sets of 30 seconds at a moderate speed then go faster and faster. Keep in mind the 3 S's (page 18) as a way to increase resistance. You should be able to recover in 30–60 seconds before you do the next set. Some people prefer to do a complete series of all the exercises and then repeat the whole sequence again, or target one area before moving on to the next (e.g., 3 sets of chest, then 3 sets of shoulders, etc.).

You can even design a circuit in which you move across the pool doing one exercise for 30 seconds, then move across to the other side doing another exercise and so on. Note that if you're doing a land-based weight-training program, there's no need to do resistance training in an aquatic environment.

Perform a Cool-Down

Stretching and cooling down after your water workout is as important to your exercise routine as

- Stretch to the point of mild tension and try to hold for 10–60 seconds. *Don't bounce.*
- Repeat all stretches 1–3 times (depending on your abilities). Each time you stretch, try to go a bit farther, if possible.
- If any stretch hurts, stop! Listen to your body, and trust your ability to distinguish between pain and a good stretch.

The Exercises

This book features exercises that target various areas so that you can get a well-rounded workout entirely in the pool. The exercises are grouped into the following series: warm-up, upper body, lower body, cardiovascular conditioning, deep-water and stretches.

The *warm-up series* is composed of gentle movements that will increase your core temperature and prepare your muscles for motion.

The *upper-body series* serves to enhance upper body strength and endurance. The secret is engaging the three S's: speed, size and shape. By playing with these variables, you can adapt the resistance so that it suits your goals. Try your best to perform each exercise through the complete range of motion at a moderate level of intensity.

Although you can certainly perform exercises without props, different types of variable resistance-training devices, or VRTDs, are available to increase the challenge. I prefer equipment that provides resistance in both directions, such as firm, rigid, plastic paddles as opposed to Styrofoam devices that assist you by floating back to the surface.

The *lower-body series* can be performed while standing next to the pool wall or away from the wall, unsupported. The legs are an important aspect of functional fitness and sports performance— some cardiovascular experts even call the legs your second heart. The legs have four major muscle groups:

- The quadriceps, or quads (the fronts of the upper legs)—responsible for lower-leg extension and the prime players in getting up from a chair.
- The hamstrings (the backs of the upper legs)—responsible for lower-leg flexion and power.
- The calves, aka gastrocnemius and soleus (the backs of the lower legs)—responsible for coming up on the balls of the feet (plantar flexion).
- The shin muscles, or anterior tibialis (the fronts of the lower legs)—responsible for pulling up the front of the foot.

The exercises in this book address all of them.

The *cardiovascular conditioning series* can be done in one place, without much pool space, or you can move across the pool while performing the movements. You choose the intensity of the work. The goal is to do each exercise series for 5 minutes; aim to perform a 30- to 40-minute aerobic session three to five times a week.

The *deep-water series* can be used as either a strenuous total-body workout or as a tool for relaxation and reflection. If you've ever tread water for any period of time, you have an idea of how great a deep-water workout can be. Similarly, if you've ever placed an innertube around your belly and just floated, you understand how relaxing a deep-water relaxation session can be. Many sports medicine experts recommend deep-water exercise as a rehabilitation method or cross-training technique since the body is allowed to recover while the cardiovascular system undergoes a high level of conditioning.

There are many methods in which you can engage in deep-water exercise. You can just go into the portion of the pool where your feet don't touch the floor

AN EXTRA CHALLENGE

If you want to challenge yourself more, cup your hands when moving your arms or place resistance devices on your hands and ankles.

If you're recovering from an injury such as ankle sprain or a pulled muscle, consider using the following approach recommended by some athletic trainers.

- Start with deep-water running/walking, jogging in place or on a tether.
- Transition slowly to shallower water.
- Continue with shallow water running with flotation devices; sprint on tether.
- Progress to shallow water with no flotation devices. Run in straight lines, progress to large circles then smaller, tighter circles, and then figure 8s in both directions.
- Return to land.

and tread water. If you're very lean and sink easily, you may find using a flotation device makes the session much safer and more enjoyable. Many options exist for flotation devices, ranging from empty milk jugs to foam noodles to aqua belts. I personally like the aqua belt because it allows for greater arm movement for a better upper-body workout. Some people who just want to focus on relaxation or moving their legs are fine with placing an inexpensive noodle under their arms, while others like to place the noodle between their legs and ride it (this allows for greater upper-body movement). I prefer placing the noodle in front of my chest and under my arms; this prevents me from getting tilted face forward into the pool (this may sound funny but it can definitely be life threatening). If you choose to do deep-water exercise untethered, you'll need to combine arm motions that return you to the starting location.

Remember, deep-water exercise is not for the non-swimmer. Just because you have a flotation device does not make up for being a non-swimmer. Also, make sure you know how to get your feet back down on the bottom of the pool. I've had many a student tell me they can swim, but they were so floatable (chubby) that they were like a cork and couldn't get their feet back down—pretty scary! So please be safe.

The *stretching series*, designed to improve flexibility and prevent injury, is best done at the end of a workout, although some people like performing a few gentle stretches after a warm-up. The choice is yours—listen to your body.

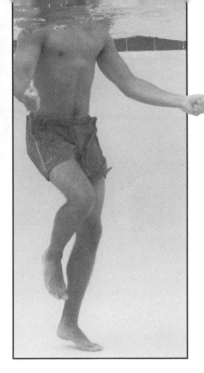

sample water workouts

Here are some workouts to get you started. Consider them suggestions. If any move doesn't feel good, try a different angle or a different exercise—your body will tell you what's right for you if you listen. The first thing you may notice when you go through one of these workouts is the omission of repetitions (reps) and sets. Unfortunately, most of us are still dialed into the outdated mindset of "How many do you want me to do, Coach?"

When deciding how many reps or sets of these exercises to do, the key is to forget about the number of reps you need to do and, instead, focus on maintaining proper posture and engaging the targeted muscles. You'll get better results by tuning in to your body and performing the movements with correct biomechanical form.

If that concept is too far out for you, start with 3–5 reps for active movements or 10 seconds for static positions. As the movement becomes easy, add more reps or think of other methods to challenge yourself. Aim to increase the number of reps to 30 or hold static poses for 30–60 seconds. Remember, more is not

necessarily better. Also, when performing the movements, focus on breathing and being centered.

(For more information on designing your own personalized routine, please turn to page 20.) Now turn on some music and enjoy the freedom a total-body water workout affords you!

general fitness

This routine is designed for an entry-level person looking for a total-body workout. It allows you to move in a pain-free manner. Don't force a move; if it doesn't feel good, don't do it. After class you shouldn't feel any worse than when you started. If you do, back off a bit next time but don't quit.

WARM-UP

EXERCISE	PAGE	DURATION
Water Walking	50	1 minute
Sideways Walking	51	1 minute
Skipping	52	1 minute

CARDIOVASCULAR CONDITIONING

High Steps with Breaststroke Arms	75 / 67	3–5 minutes
High Steps with Fly Arms	75 / 69	3–5 minutes
High Steps with Punching	75 / 70	3–5 minutes
Jumping Jacks with Jumping Jack Arms: Side	76 / 74	3–5 minutes
Jumping Jacks with Punching	76 / 70	3–5 minutes
Cross-Country Skiing with Cross-Country Arms	77 / 71	3–5 minutes

UPPER-BODY CONDITIONING

EXERCISE	PAGE	DURATION
Chest Press	53	30 seconds
Lateral Raise	55	30 seconds
Chest Tap	57	30 seconds

LOWER-BODY CONDITIONING

Forward Leg Raise	59	30 seconds
Side Leg Raise	62	30 seconds
Heel Raise	65	30 seconds

STRETCHING

Hamstring Stretch	93	30 seconds
Calf Stretch	93	30 seconds
Elbow Touches	95	30 seconds

advanced general conditioning

You can try this routine if you're relatively fit, injury-free and/or proficient in water exercise.

WARM-UP

EXERCISE	PAGE	DURATION
Water Walking	50	1 minute
Sideways Walking	51	1 minute
Skipping	52	1 minute

CARDIOVASCULAR CONDITIONING

EXERCISE	PAGE	DURATION
Cross-Country Skiing with Jumping Jack Arms: Side	77 / 74	1–5 minutes
Cross-Country Skiing with Piston Arms	77 / 69	1–5 minutes
Straight-Leg Kicks with Breaststroke Arms	78 / 67	1–5 minutes
Straight-Leg Kicks with Paddlewheels	78 / 72	1–5 minutes
Soccer Kicks with Hug Arms	79 / 68	1–5 minutes
Soccer Kicks with Fly Arms	79 / 69	1–5 minutes
Rock Around the World (deep-water)	92	1–5 minutes
6 o'clock to 12 o'clock Jumps	83	1–5 minutes
9 o'clock to 3 o'clock Jumps	84	1–5 minutes
High Steps with Paddlewheels	75 / 72	1–5 minutes

UPPER-BODY CONDITIONING

EXERCISE	PAGE	DURATION
Frontal Raise	56	1 minute
Washboard	58	1 minute
Punching	70	1 minute
Chest Tap	57	1 minute

LOWER-BODY CONDITIONING

Leg Curl	63	1 minute
Forward Leg Raise	59	1 minute
Backward Leg Raise	60	1 minute
Side Leg Raise	62	1 minute
Leg Extension	64	1 minute
Rocking Horse	81	1 minute

STRETCHING

Hamstring Stretch	93	30 seconds
Calf Stretch	93	30 seconds
Elbow Touches	95	30 seconds

sports conditioning

This routine is designed for those who like to challenge themselves, are cross-training or are recovering from a sports injury.

WARM-UP		
EXERCISE	**PAGE**	**DURATION**
Water Walking	50	1 minute
Sideways Walking	51	1 minute
Skipping	52	1 minute
Jump Rope	85	1 minute

CARDIOVASCULAR CONDITIONING *do three sets*		
High Steps with Chest Tap Arms	75 / 73	15–30 seconds
High Steps with Jumping Jack Arms: Frontal	75 / 74	15–30 seconds
High Steps with Washboard Arms	75 / 68	15–30 seconds
High Steps with Arm Circles each direction	75 / 71	15–30 seconds
Underwater Rockets	82	15–30 seconds
Cross-Country Skiing with Fly Arms	77 / 69	15–30 seconds
Cross-Country Skiing with Cross-Country Arms	77 / 71	15–30 seconds
Soccer Kicks with Jumping Jack Arms: Side	79 / 74	15–30 seconds

UPPER-BODY CONDITIONING *do three sets, max intensity*

EXERCISE	PAGE	DURATION
Punching	70	1 minute
Fly	54	1 minute
Chest Tap	57	1 minute
Lateral Raise	55	1 minute
Washboard	58	1 minute
Frontal Raise	56	1 minute

LOWER-BODY CONDITIONING *do three sets, max intensity*

Straight-Leg Kicks	78	1 minute
Butt Kickers	80	1 minute
Soccer Kicks	79	1 minute
Heel Raise	65	1 minute
Toe Lift	66	1 minute
Side Leg Raise	62	1 minute

COOL-DOWN AND STRETCHING

Water Walking	50	5–10 min
Sideways Walking	51	5–10 min
Skipping	52	5–10 min
Hamstring Stretch	93	hold 30 seconds
Calf Stretch	93	hold 30 seconds
Elbow Touches	95	hold 30 seconds

deep-water workout

This routine can be ideal for people with joint considerations or it can be very challenging for the elite athlete. It's an excellent way to cross-train between difficult land-based activities like basketball, running or tennis. The critical elements are intensity and duration.

This method allows you to keep your aerobic fitness high and your joint trauma low. Some people like to attach themselves to a solid object and do their deep-water workout in place, while others like the moving around in the pool and then returning to the starting location. You might consider the support of an inexpensive noodle or an aqua belt.

If you want to challenge your upper body more, wear aqua gloves; you can even place ankle cuffs on your legs for additional resistance. There's no right or wrong way—just start moving! Try to work out for 20–40 minutes. However, be careful when doing any deep-water routine because drowning is possible. *CAUTION:* If you can't swim, do NOT try this routine.

WARM-UP

EXERCISE	PAGE	DURATION
Water Walking	50	3–5 minutes
Sideways Walking	51	3–5 minutes
Skipping	52	3–5 minutes

CARDIOVASCULAR CONDITIONING *repeat as desired*

Deep-Water Jogging	86	3–5 minutes
Straight-Leg Kicks (deep-water)	88	3–5 minutes
Soccer Kicks (deep-water)	89	3–5 minutes
Cross-Country Skiing (deep-water)	87	3–5 minutes
Deep-Water Sit-Ups	90	3–5 minutes
Twist (deep-water)	91	3–5 minutes
Rock Around the World (deep-water)	92	3–5 minutes

COOL-DOWN

Water Walking	50	3–5 minutes
Sideways Walking	51	3–5 minutes
Skipping	52	3–5 minutes

arthritis

The key to exercise for people with arthritis is to maintain range of motion (joint flexibility). The old saying regarding exercise and arthritis is "*motion is lotion.*" Water workouts are ideal as therapy because water can minimize the pain and can assist in possible improvement of range of motion. Below is a list of common guidelines for persons with arthritis as suggested by medical doctors and physical therapists.

- Never exercise unless following the advice of a health care professional.
- Don't over-exercise.
- Don't neglect your medical routine.
- Don't mask pain by over-medicating.
- Don't exercise a "hot joint" (a joint that's swollen or warm to the touch).
- Obey the two-hour rule: If you hurt more two hours post-exercise, you did too much. Do less next time.

Be gentle and start slowly. Perform this workout only as tolerated.

WARM-UP		
EXERCISE	**PAGE**	**DURATION**
Water Walking	50	as needed or tolerated
Sideways Walking	51	as needed or tolerated
LOWER-BODY CONDITIONING		
Leg Extension	64	as needed or tolerated
Side Leg Raise	62	as needed or tolerated
Toe Lift	66	as needed or tolerated
1-2-3 Leg Raise & Hold	61	as needed or tolerated

UPPER-BODY CONDITIONING

EXERCISE	PAGE	DURATION
Hula Hands	72	as needed or tolerated
Breaststroke Arms	67	as needed or tolerated
Frontal Raise	56	as needed or tolerated
Arm Curls	73	as needed or tolerated

CARDIOVASCULAR CONDITIONING

High Steps with Hula Hands	75 / 72	as needed or tolerated
Cross-Country Skiing with Arm Curls	77 / 73	as needed or tolerated
Leg Curl with Frontal Raise	63 / 56	as needed or tolerated

STRETCHING

Calf Stretch	93	as needed or tolerated
Shoulder Stretch	96	as needed or tolerated
Elbow Touches	95	as needed or tolerated
Wrist Stretches	97	as needed or tolerated
Lower Back Stretch	98	as needed or tolerated

frozen shoulder

A frozen shoulder usually results from non-use of the shoulder because of a painful shoulder condition such as tendinitis or bursitis. If the arm isn't used for a period of time, adhesions may form on the sleeve-like structure that holds the ball and socket portion of the shoulder joint together. If the shoulder isn't moved for two to three weeks, these adhesions will become very dense and strong and will result in a shoulder that can't move freely—or, frozen shoulder. Water will minimize the pain and possibly improve range of motion. If a shoulder hasn't been used for a long period of time, a health care professional should be consulted. For more information, see one of my other books, *Healthy Shoulder Handbook* (Ulysses Press, 2010).

Caution: Avoid forceful arm movements or extreme range of motion; move arms slowly through full range of motion under the water.

WARM-UP

EXERCISE	PAGE	DURATION
Sideways Walking	51	as needed or tolerated
Cross-Country Skiing	77	as needed or tolerated

UPPER-BODY CONDITIONING

EXERCISE	PAGE	DURATION
Chest Tap	57	as needed or tolerated
Hula Hands	72	as needed or tolerated
Arm Curls	73	as needed or tolerated
Paddlewheels	72	as needed or tolerated

STRETCHING

EXERCISE	PAGE	DURATION
Elbow Touches	95	as needed or tolerated
Double Wood Chop	96	as needed or tolerated
Shoulder Stretch	96	as needed or tolerated

low back pain

Low back pain is caused by a variety of sources—weak abdominals, tight hamstrings and quadriceps, improper body mechanics, poor posture, overuse, facet and joint problems, and herniated discs. Many arm movements, such as overhead reaching and arm extension, affect the low back. Vertical jumping can also bother those with low back issues. Some water exercisers injure their backs when they do lateral leg raises and lean too much at the waist; the leg should only be raised 45–50°, the toes should point forward and the trunk should be stabilized and not move.

Exercises that strengthen the abdominals and stretch the hamstrings as well as the low back muscles are recommended. If you have a back problem, good neutral spine technique is especially important. Avoid using leg and ankle weights, as well as hand paddles that cause you to "feel it" in your low back. Here are other tips for a safe workout:

- Keep movements fluid.
- If pain is present more than two hours post-exercise, cut back exercise duration and/or intensity.
- Avoid impact activities.
- Perform exercises in warm water (82–92°F) if possible.
- Try to move through full range of motion and, if possible, keep it pain free.
- Listen to your body.

WARM-UP

EXERCISE	PAGE	DURATION
Water Walking	50	as needed or tolerated
Sideways Walking	51	as needed or tolerated

LOWER-BODY CONDITIONING

Leg Extension	64	as needed or tolerated
Side Leg Raise	62	as needed or tolerated
Heel Raise	65	as needed or tolerated

UPPER-BODY CONDITIONING

Lateral Raise	55	as needed or tolerated
Chest Tap	57	as needed or tolerated
Fly	54	as needed or tolerated

CARDIOVASCULAR CONDITIONING

Deep-Water Jogging	86	as needed or tolerated
Cross-Country Skiing (deep-water)	87	as needed or tolerated

STRETCHING

Lower Back Stretch	98	as needed or tolerated
Calf Stretch	93	as needed or tolerated
Hamstring Stretch	93	as needed or tolerated

hip

Although the hip is the powerhouse of the body, many conditions (from bursitis to arthritis to athletic injuries) can affect the joint. Deep-water exercise is a great way to improve range of motion without inducing trauma.

WARM-UP

EXERCISE	PAGE	DURATION
Water Walking	50	as needed or tolerated
Sideways Walking	51	as needed or tolerated

LOWER-BODY CONDITIONING

EXERCISE	PAGE	DURATION
Forward Leg Raise	59	as needed or tolerated
Leg Curl	63	as needed or tolerated
Deep-Water Jogging	86	as needed or tolerated
Cross-Country Skiing (deep-water)	87	as needed or tolerated

STRETCHING

EXERCISE	PAGE	DURATION
Calf Stretch	93	as needed or tolerated
Lower Back Stretch	98	as needed or tolerated
Hamstring Stretch	93	as needed or tolerated

knee

If you have knee issues, it's a good idea to keep "soft knees" when doing a water workout. Additionally, avoid twisting your body with your feet planted; the knees and toes should *always* point in the same direction. Performing very wide jumping jacks or jumping and landing without bending the knees to absorb the load can aggravate knee problems. Also, any exercise that uses the quadriceps forcefully, such as leg extensions, can trigger knee pain. Remember: Force rather than speed is better when doing leg exercises. Another precaution is to avoid overflexion of the knee joint when doing quadriceps stretches (i.e., bringing the heel toward the buttocks). Practice learning how to jump and land correctly.

WARM-UP

EXERCISE	PAGE	DURATION
Water Walking	50	as needed or tolerated
Sideways Walking	51	as needed or tolerated

LOWER-BODY CONDITIONING

Side Leg Raise	62	as needed or tolerated
Forward Leg Raise	59	as needed or tolerated
Cross-Country Skiing	77	as needed or tolerated
High Steps	75	as needed or tolerated

STRETCHING

Calf Stretch	93	as needed or tolerated
Ankle Circles	94	as needed or tolerated

shin splints

Shin splints refer to the pain that occurs in the front of the lower leg when the connective tissue pulls away from the bone. Running or aerobic dancing on hard surfaces can contribute to shin splints. Anatomical abnormalities of the foot, as well as strength and flexibility imbalances in the lower leg muscles, can also result in shin splints.

WARM-UP

EXERCISE	PAGE	DURATION
Sideways Walking	51	as needed or tolerated

LOWER-BODY CONDITIONING

Heel Raise	65	as needed or tolerated
Toe Lift	66	as needed or tolerated

CARDIOVASCULAR CONDITIONING

Deep-Water Jogging	86	as needed or tolerated
Cross-Country Skiing (deep-water)	87	as needed or tolerated

STRETCHING

Ankle Circles	94	as needed or tolerated
Calf Stretch	93	as needed or tolerated
Heel Raise	65	as needed or tolerated
Toe Lift	66	as needed or tolerated

ankle/feet

Even though injuries to the ankles and feet are greatly reduced in the water, it's important to pay attention to the way you land to avoid supination and pronation problems. There are several ways to lessen the impact on the feet: working in deeper water, wearing aquatic shoes (which also protect the bottoms of the feet), wearing an aqua-jogger while performing suspended deep-water exercises. Use caution with range-of-motion and strengthening moves until any swelling/pain subsides—don't overstretch. Gradually increase weight bearing. People with diabetes need to pay attention to drying their feet completely; consider using a hair dryer to blow-dry between the toes.

WARM-UP

EXERCISE	PAGE	DURATION
Ankle Circles	94	as needed or tolerated
Calf Stretch	93	as needed or tolerated
Water Walking	50	as needed or tolerated
Sideways Walking	51	as needed or tolerated
Forward Leg Raise	59	as needed or tolerated

LOWER-BODY CONDITIONING

Heel Raise	65	as needed or tolerated
Toe Lift	66	as needed or tolerated
1-2-3 Leg Raise & Hold	61	as needed or tolerated
Straight-Leg Kicks	78	as needed or tolerated

STRETCHING

Calf Stretch	93	as needed or tolerated
Ankle Circles	94	as needed or tolerated

freeflow routine 1

This routine is designed for people who like to express their creativity. Basically, select 5 of your favorite cardiovascular leg moves (pages 75–81) and 5 of your favorite arm add-ons (pages 67–74). Then turn on your music or even a clock.

1. Start with one leg move and stay with it for 5 minutes or switch at the end of every song, but switch your arm motions every minute. One example is to begin with cross-country legs and arm flies, then switch to punching, etc. Then switch to a different leg movement and use the same arm motion.
2. After 5 songs or 20–25 minutes, grab a noodle and do 4 songs' worth of deep-water moves.
3. Finish up with some upper-body strength training and a few minutes of stretching.

freeflow routine 2

This workout (and my personal favorite) is similar to the first routine, except you need enough space around you to move in every direction. Ten feet in all directions is fine. As with Routine 1, allow your body and your creativity to be the guide. I like to start with jogging forward and backward with breaststroke arms, then switch to cross-country legs with jumping jack arms, etc. It's more challenging to select arm motions that counteract the direction in which you're traveling (e.g., hugging arms and forward jogging). Mix and match to meet your fancy, then try the same concept with deep-water exercises. Turn on some motivating music and go with the flow!

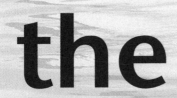

part 3
the
exercises

STARTING POSITION: Stand at a comfortable depth in the pool, ideally waist to chest deep.

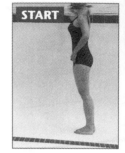

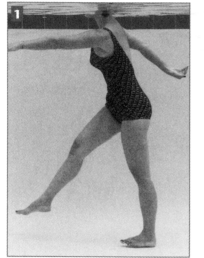

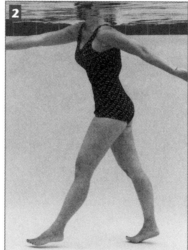

1–2 Walk back and forth across the pool, swinging your arms fully as if walking, then progress to breaststroke arm motions, keeping your arms in the water. Take both large and small strides. Depending on how you feel, you may stop at each end and perform a gentle leg stretch.

VARIATIONS: Walk on your heels. Walk on your toes.

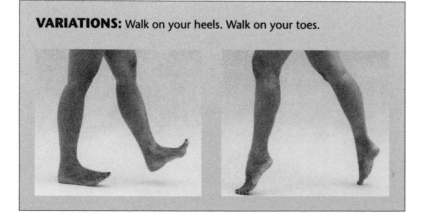

STARTING POSITION: Stand at a comfortable depth in the pool, ideally waist to chest deep.

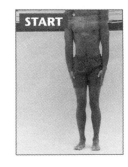
START

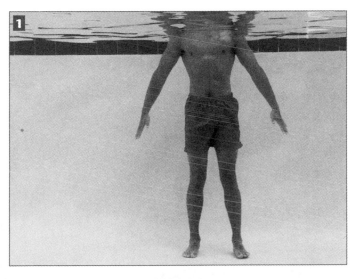
1

1–2 Walk sideways across the pool, using your arms fully to the side while keeping them underwater. Take both large and small steps.

Depending on how you feel, you may stop at each end and perform a gentle leg stretch.

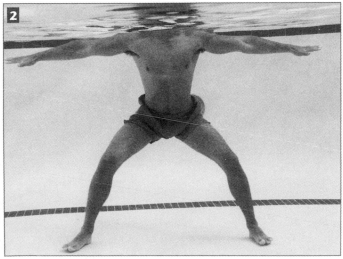
2

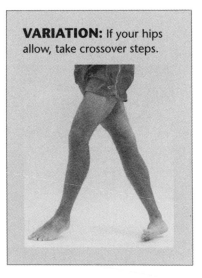
VARIATION: If your hips allow, take crossover steps.

STARTING POSITION: Stand at a comfortable depth in the pool, ideally waist to chest deep.

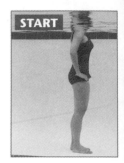

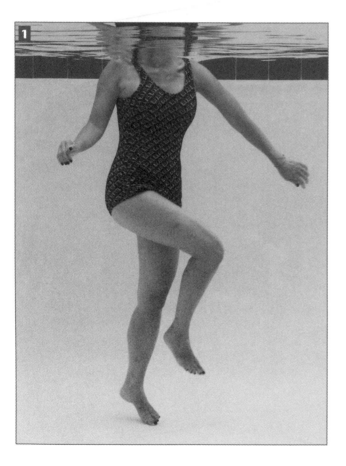

1 Skip across the pool. Use your arms any way you want to loosen up your body.

Now hop, skip and jump across the pool.

STARTING POSITION: Stand tall in a stable position (e.g., one leg forward, one leg back) and hold a VRTD in each hand at your chest, VRTD facing forward.

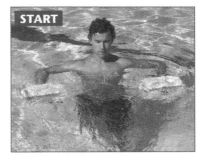

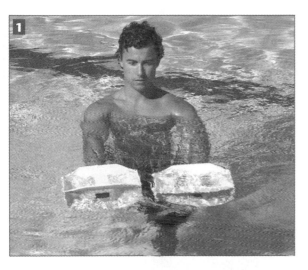

1 Push both arms forward as quickly as possible.

2 Return to starting position.

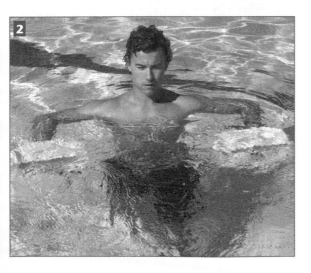

VARIATION: You can also do this one arm at a time.

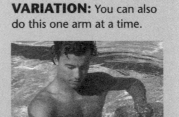

STARTING POSITION: Stand tall in a stable position (e.g., one leg forward, one leg back) and hold a VRTD in each hand. Extend both arms in front of your shoulders, palms facing each other.

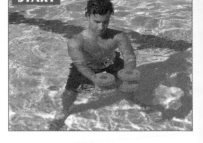

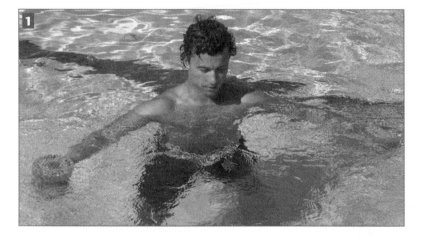

1 As quickly as possible, take your arms out to the sides.

2 Return to starting position.

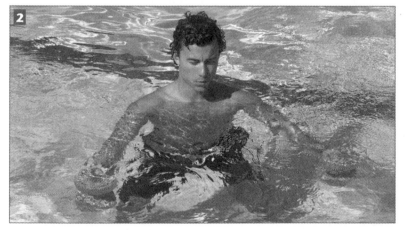

STARTING POSITION: Stand tall in a stable position (e.g., one leg forward, one leg back) and hold a VRTD in each hand, arms along your sides.

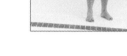

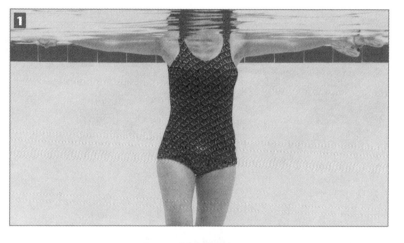

1 Lift both arms up sideways to surface level as quickly as possible.

2 Return to starting position.

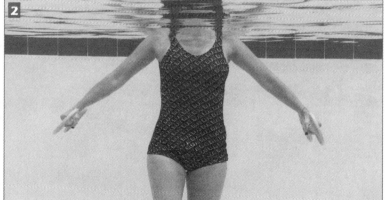

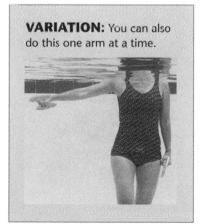

VARIATION: You can also do this one arm at a time.

STARTING POSITION: Stand tall in a stable position (e.g., one leg forward, one leg back) and hold a VRTD in each hand, arms out in front of you at shoulder height and palms facing down.

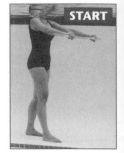

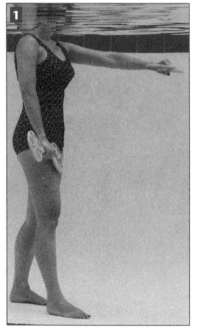

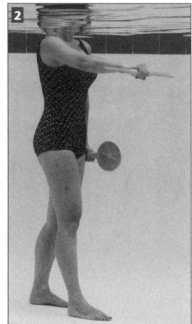

1 Push your right arm down to your thigh/hip area.

2 Bring it up to surface level as quickly as possible; when your right arm comes up, push your left arm down.

Continue alternating arms.

STARTING POSITION: Stand tall in a stable position (e.g., one leg forward, one leg back) and hold a VRTD in each hand with your arms extended out to the sides at shoulder level, palms facing forward.

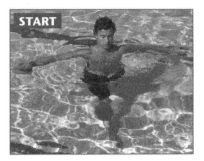

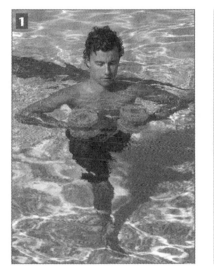

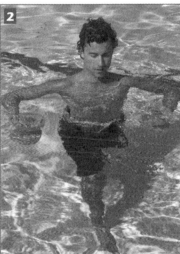

1 As quickly as possible, bend your elbows and bring your hands to your chest.

2 Return to starting position.

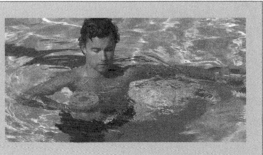

VARIATION: You can also do this one arm at a time.

washboard

target: biceps, triceps, trapezius, shoulders

STARTING POSITION: Stand tall but lean slightly forward. Hold a VRTD in each hand near your armpits.

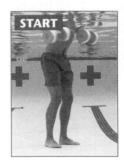

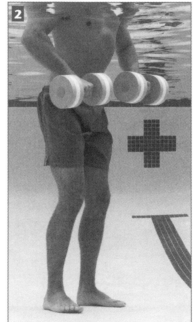

1–2 Press both arms down and up vigorously.

PISTON ARMS VARIATION: As you advance, you can move one arm down as the other arm comes up.

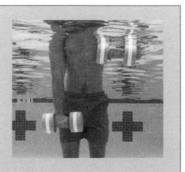

STARTING POSITION: Stand tall with proper neutral posture. You may place your hands on your hips.

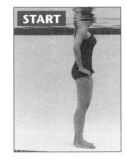

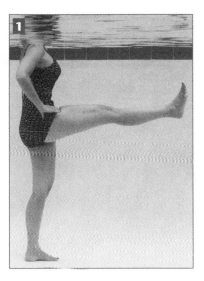

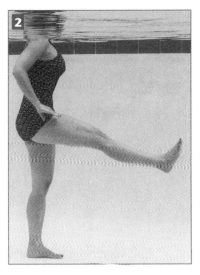

1 Keeping your right leg straight, quickly lift it straight up with your toes pointed up. You should feel this motion in your quads.

2 Keeping your lower back motionless, quickly lower your leg.

Finish your reps on this leg and then perform with your left leg.

CAUTION: If you have lower back issues, be careful not to arch your back when performing this exercise.

STARTING POSITION: Stand tall with proper neutral posture. You may place your hands on your hips.

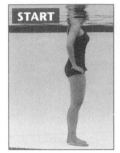

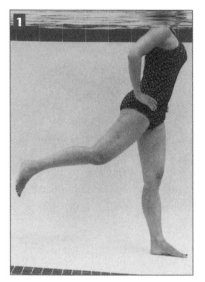

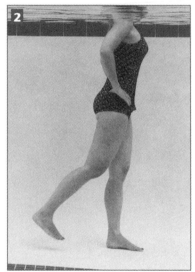

1 Keeping your right leg straight, slowly swing it backward, being mindful to engage your butt muscles.

2 Smoothly return to starting position.

Finish your reps on this leg and then perform with your left leg.

This exercise combines the movements of the Forward Leg Raise and Backward Leg Raise.

STARTING POSITION: Stand tall with proper neutral posture. You may place your hands on your hips.

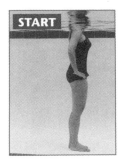

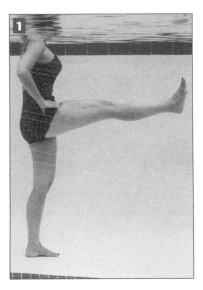

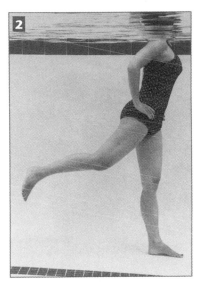

1 Keeping your right leg straight, quickly swing your leg forward with your toes pointed up. You should feel this motion in your quads.

2 Keeping your lower back motionless, quickly swing your leg backward.

Now swing it forward again and hold the position for a few seconds. Continue swinging, holding the position of the third swing. After you've performed the prescribed number of reps, switch legs.

CAUTION: Be careful if you have hip issues.

STARTING POSITION: Stand tall with proper neutral posture.

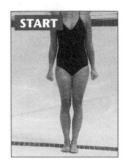

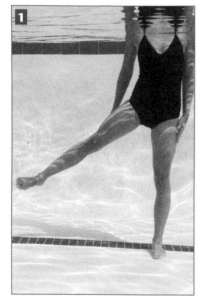

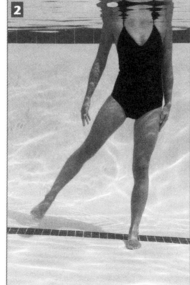

1 Keeping your right leg straight, quickly lift it out to the side. Be mindful that the motion comes from the hip joint; don't swing your leg or lean forward.

2 Quickly and smoothly return to starting position.

Finish your reps on this leg and then perform with your left leg.

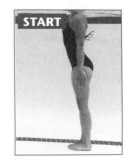

You may want to perform a hamstring stretch between sets to avoid cramps.

CAUTION: If you have lower back issues, be careful to not arch your lower back.

STARTING POSITION: Stand tall with proper neutral posture.

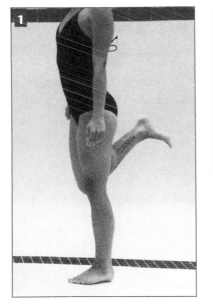

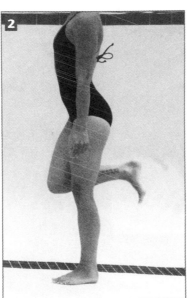

1 Keeping your foot flexed, bend your right knee to bring your right heel toward your butt as high as is comfortable.

2 Straighten your leg again.

Finish your reps on this leg and then perform with your left leg.

CAUTION: Be careful not to snap the knee joint nor hyperextend the knee.

STARTING POSITION: Stand tall with proper neutral posture and place your hands on your hips.

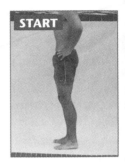

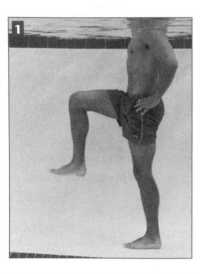

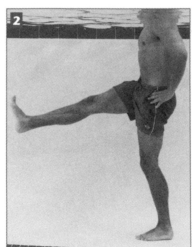

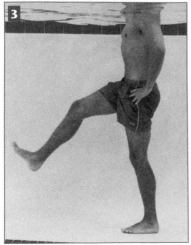

1 Bending your right knee to 90°, raise it to waist height or whatever is comfortable.

2 Extend your leg straight out, but don't force the motion.

3 Curl your leg back to the starting position.

Finish your reps on this leg and then perform with your left leg.

CAUTION: Stay mindful of cramps. It's recommended that you stretch the calf muscles between sets.

STARTING POSITION: Stand tall with proper neutral posture and your feet together.

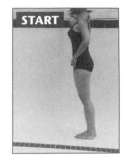

1 Keeping your feet together, come up on the balls of your feet.

Lower to starting position.

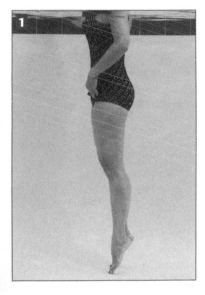

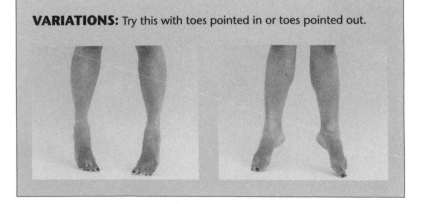

VARIATIONS: Try this with toes pointed in or toes pointed out.

This exercise is excellent for people who have foot drop and bouts of shin splints.

STARTING POSITION: Stand tall with proper neutral posture.

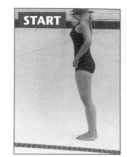

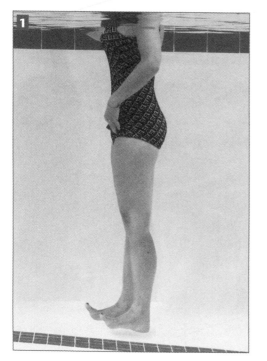

1 Slowly rock back onto your heels, lifting the fronts of your feet off the pool floor. Hold for several seconds.

Lower to starting position.

cardiovascular conditioning

This cardiovascular section is arranged menu style, allowing you to mix and match upper-body motions with different lower-body movements for an endless variety of exercises. Generally when I teach a class, I have the class do the same leg motions for about 5 minutes and change the arm motions every minute. This approach keeps the exercise from getting monotonous and prevents muscle fatigue. For a full 40-minute workout, start with high steps (page 75) and move through the leg movements, ending with the jumping sequence. The goal is to do each movement for 5 minutes at the intensity of your choice. When you get to the jumping sequence, do each jump for 1 minute. Each movement includes recommended arm variations; you can do these or pick others from the arm add-ons menu (pages 67–74). For a quick warm-up, pick any of the lower-body movements (pages 75–81) and pair it with a few upper-body motions.

arm add-ons

breaststroke arms   *target: upper back*

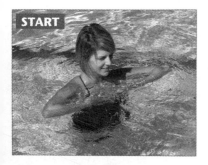

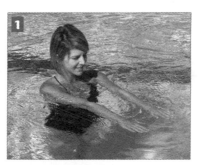

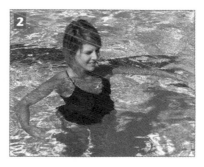

STARTING POSITION: Hold your hands at your chest.

1–2 Extend your arms forward then pull the

water into your sides as if doing a breaststroke.

hug arms

target: biceps

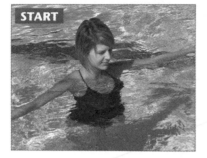

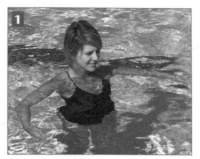

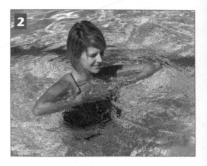

STARTING POSITION: Raise your arms to shoulder height and bring them out to the sides so that they're parallel to the floor.

1–2 Scoop your arms in toward your chest as if hugging someone.

Continue scooping water in toward your chest.

washboard arms

target: biceps, triceps, trapezius, shoulders

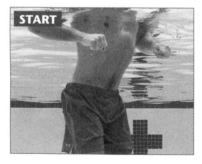

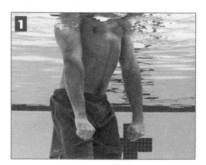

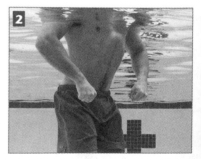

STARTING POSITION: Hold your hands near your armpits.

1–2 Press both arms down and up vigorously.

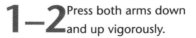

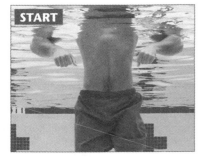 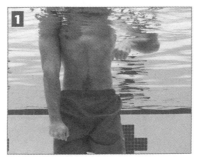 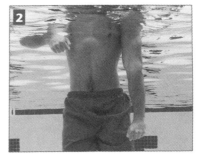

STARTING POSITION: Hold your hands near your armpits.

1–2 Press your right arm down. As you bring your right arm up, simultaneously press your left arm down.

fly arms — *target: chest, upper back*

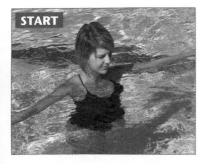 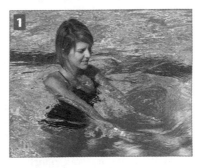

STARTING POSITION: Extend your arms straight out to the sides at shoulder height.

1 Keeping your arms straight, clap your hands together quickly in front of your body.

Return to starting position.

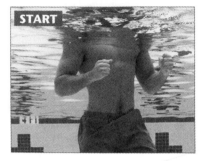

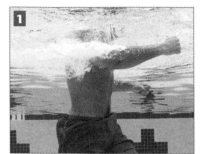

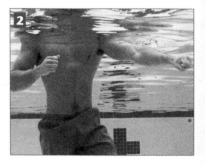

STARTING POSITION: Hold your hands at your chest.

1–2 Extend one arm forward then bring it back to your chest as the other arm punches forward.

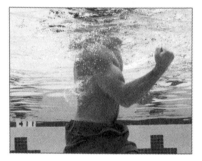

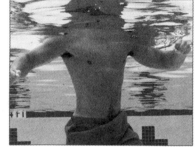

3–4 You can also perform uppercuts, roundhouses, or jabs.

VARIATION: Punch with both arms simultaneously. For additional cardio work, punch with vigor.

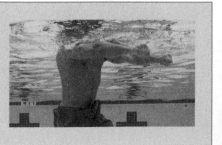

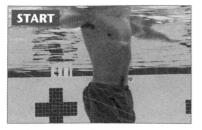

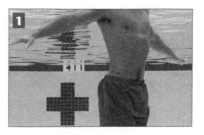

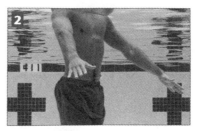

STARTING POSITION: Extend your arms straight out to the sides at shoulder height, keeping them underwater.

1–2 Keeping your arms straight, make small circles forward then progress to larger and faster arm circles.

Reverse direction.

cross-country arms — *target: shoulders*

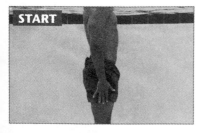

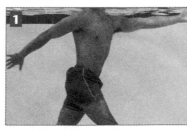

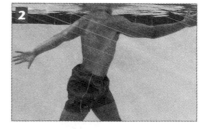

STARTING POSITION: Rest your arms along your sides.

1–2 Keeping your arms somewhat straight, pump your arms back and forth as if you had a ski pole in each hand. One arm should move forward as the other moves backward.

To increase resistance, cup your hands. To decrease resistance, slice through the water.

arm add-ons

paddlewheels

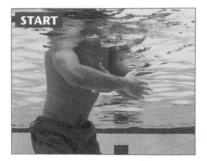

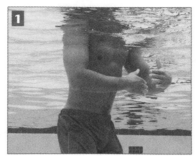

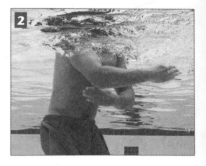

STARTING POSITION: Bend your arms 90 degrees with your arms in front of your chest approximately shoulder height.

1–2 Moving only from your elbows, circle your arms forward.

Reverse direction.

hula hands

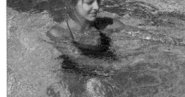

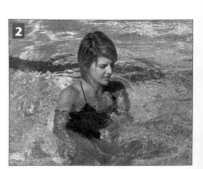

STARTING POSITION: Extend your arms straight out in front of you at shoulder height.

1–2 Move your arms and hands as if you're doing a hula dance, keeping your arms straight but soft. Be creative

with the arm motions—notice the difference in resistance.

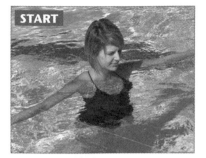 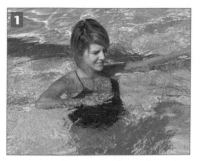 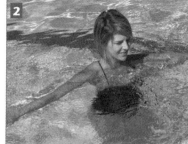

STARTING POSITION: Extend your arms straight out to the sides at shoulder height.

1–2 Bending your arms at the elbow, tap yourself on the chest, alternating hands.

arm curls   *target: biceps, triceps*

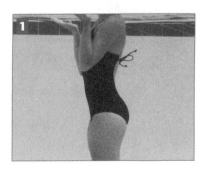 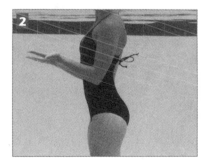

STARTING POSITION: Rest your arms along your sides.

1 With open hands, bring your right hand toward your right shoulder and your left hand toward your left shoulder.

2 Lower your arms and repeat quickly.

arm add-ons

jumping jack arms: side
target: shoulders (lateral)

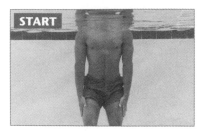

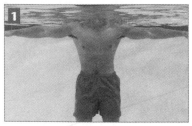

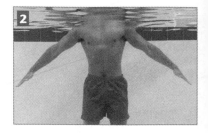

STARTING POSITION: Rest your arms along your sides.

1–2 Keeping your arms straight, quickly lift your arms sideways to the surface of the water. Keep your arms underwater—you get the

resistance from the water, not the air.

Quickly return to starting position and repeat.

jumping jack arms: frontal
target: shoulders (frontal)

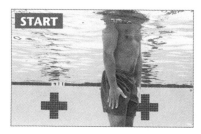

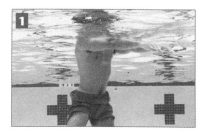

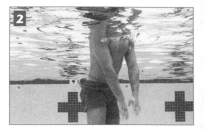

STARTING POSITION: Rest your arms along your sides.

1–2 Keeping your arms straight, quickly lift them forward to the surface of the water. Keep your arms underwater—you get the

resistance from the water, not the air.

Quickly return to starting position and repeat.

VARIATION: You can do this one arm at a time. Raise one arm to the surface of the water; as you lower the raised arm, simultaneously bring the other one up.

Perform leg movements for 5 minutes; change arm movements every 60 seconds.

STARTING POSITION: Stand tall with proper neutral posture.

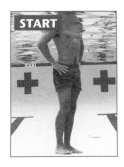

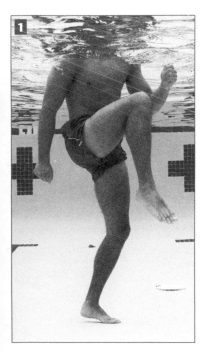

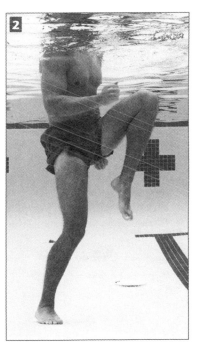

1–2 Lift your knees high as if stepping on a chair; try to get your heels to the pool floor periodically to avoid calf cramps. Add arms (see variations below) as desired.

RECOMMENDED ARM VARIATIONS: Punching (page 70), Paddlewheels (page 72)

jumping jacks
target: aerobic fitness, inner/outer leg endurance

Perform leg movements for 5 minutes; change arm movements every 60 seconds.

STARTING POSITION: Stand tall with your feet together and arms by your sides.

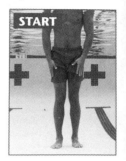

1 Jump up and spread your legs a comfortable distance, approximately shoulder-width apart. Add arms (see variations below) as desired.

2 Return your legs to starting position and continue jumping.

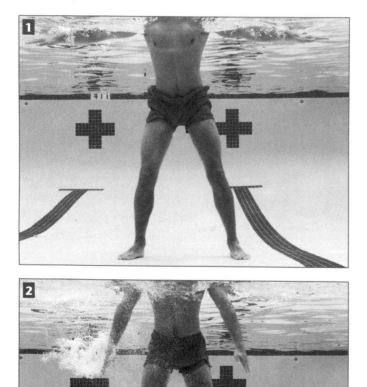

RECOMMENDED ARM VARIATIONS: Jumping Jack Arms: Side (page 74), Jumping Jack Arms: Frontal (page 74), Fly Arms (page 69)

Perform leg movements for 5 minutes; change arm movements every 60 seconds.

CAUTION: Be careful not to lunge farther than is comfortable as this could trigger lower back pain and knee discomfort.

STARTING POSITION: Stand tall with your arms along your sides.

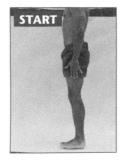

1 Jump up and move one leg forward and the other leg backward a comfortable distance. Add arms (see variations below) as desired.

2 Continue alternating leg motions.

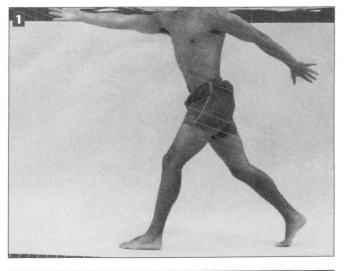

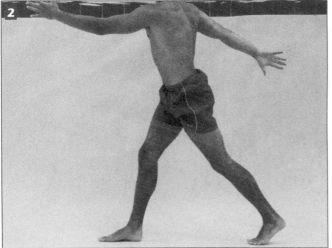

RECOMMENDED ARM VARIATIONS: Breaststroke Arms (page 67), Cross-Country Arms (page 71), Arm Curls (page 73)

78 | **straight-leg kicks** | *target: quadriceps, hamstrings*

Perform leg movements for 5 minutes; change arm movements every 60 seconds.

STARTING POSITION: Stand tall with your hands on your hips.

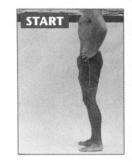
START

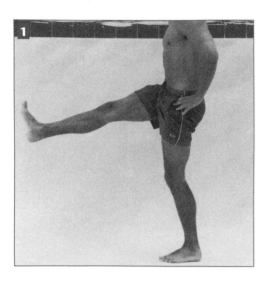
1

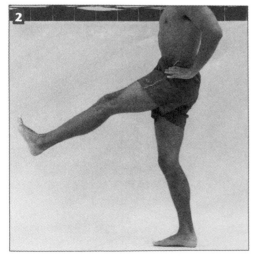
2

1 Quickly lift your right leg straight up to the front; be careful not to kick too high. Add arms (see variations below) as desired.

2 Alternating quickly, bring your right leg down and lift your left.

RECOMMENDED ARM VARIATIONS: Jumping Jack Arms: Side (page 74), right hand to left leg and vice versa

Perform leg movements for 5 minutes; change arm movements every 60 seconds.

STARTING POSITION: Stand tall with your hands on your hips.

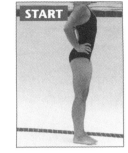

1–2 Lift your right knee and extend your leg as if kicking someone in the rear; be careful not to lock out your knee or kick too high. Add arms (see variations below) as desired.

Bring your leg down and quickly kick with the other leg.

RECOMMENDED ARM VARIATIONS: Chest Tap Arms (page 73), Arm Circles (page 71)

leg movements

butt kickers

target: aerobic fitness, hamstrings

Perform leg movements for 5 minutes; change arm movements every 60 seconds.

CAUTION: People with knee issues should only bend to 90°.

STARTING POSITION: Stand tall with your arms alongside your body.

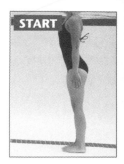

1 Flex/curl your right leg toward your bottom. Be careful not to curl your leg too high or you might get a hamstring cramp.

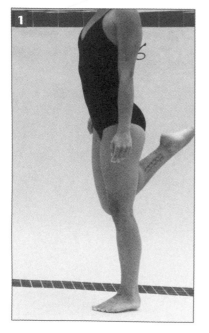

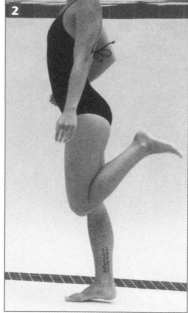

2 Return to starting position and perform with your left leg.

Continue alternating legs, adding arms (see variations below) as desired.

RECOMMENDED ARM VARIATIONS: Arm Curls (page 73), Fly Arms (page 69)

Perform leg movements for 5 minutes; change arm movements every 60 seconds.

STARTING POSITION: Stand tall with your left leg forward and right leg back.

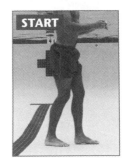

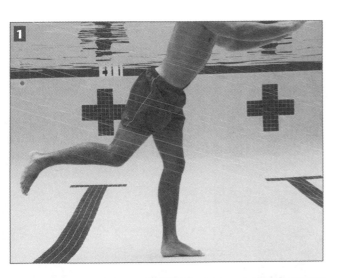

1–2 Rock forward on to your left leg then immediately rock back to your right leg—the movement should be fluid and smooth. Add arms (see variations below) as desired.

Continue rocking back and forth for 1 minute then move the right leg to the forward position.

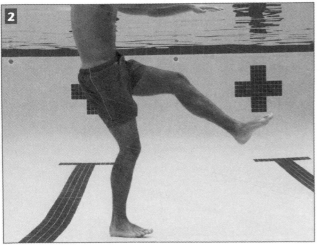

RECOMMENDED ARM VARIATIONS: Breaststroke Arms (page 67), Hug Arms (page 68), Jumping Jack Arms: Side (page 74)

STARTING POSITION: Stand with your shoulders under the water, knees slightly bent.

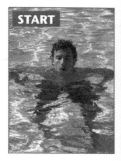

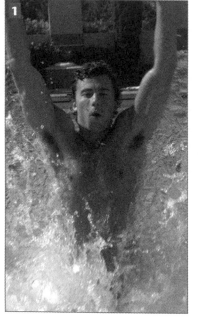

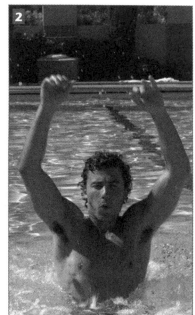

1–2 Jump up and down as high as you can for 1 minute.

STARTING POSITION: Stand with proper neutral posture, knees slightly bent. You can place your hands on your hips if you like. Imagine you're at the 6 o'clock position of a clock.

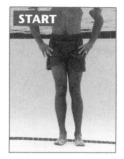

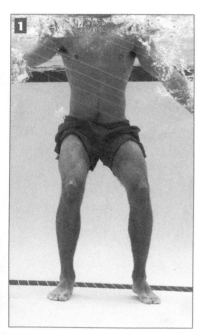

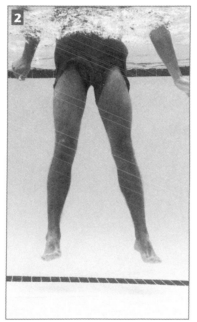

1–2 Jump forward to 12 o'clock (you decide how far forward to jump). Without pausing, jump back to 6 o'clock.

Continue for 1 minute.

RECOMMENDED ARM VARIATIONS: Breaststroke Arms (page 67) as you pull forward, Hug Arms (page 68) as you go back, Jumping Jack Arms to the front and sides (page 74)

STARTING POSITION: Stand tall with proper neutral posture and place your hands on your hips. Imagine you're at the 9 o'clock position of a clock.

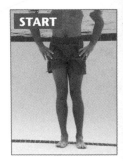

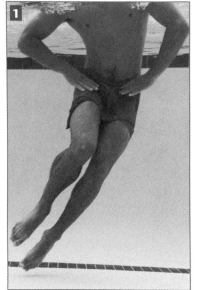

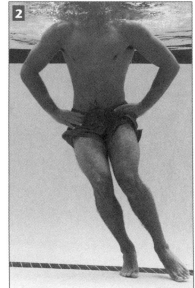

1–2 Jump over to 3 o'clock (you decide how far sideward to jump). Without pausing, jump back to 9 o'clock.

Continue for 1 minute.

RECOMMENDED ARM VARIATIONS: Jumping Jack Arms: Side (page 74), Chest Tap Arms (page 73), Arm Curls (page 73)

STARTING POSITION: Stand tall with your arms by your sides and hands in fists.

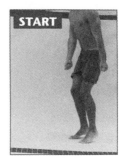

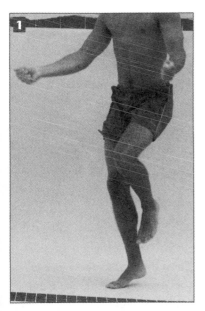

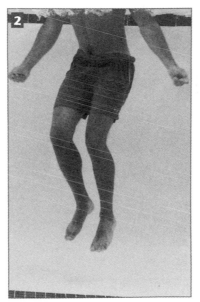

1 Pretend to skip rope by alternating one leg then the other.

Continue for 1 minute.

2 Pretend to jump rope with both feet together, jumping as high as you want.

Continue for 1 minute.

STARTING POSITION: With your feet off the bottom of the pool with or without a flotation device and with or without a tethered attachment, lean slightly forward.

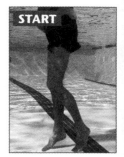

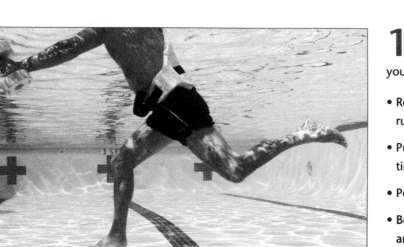

1–2 Move your legs as if jogging and pump your arms as follows:

- Really pump your arms as if running up a hill.

- Punch one arm forward at a time and really recoil it back.

- Perform arm curls.

- Be creative—move your arms any way you wish.

- If you're untethered, use your arm motions to allow you to move a few feet forward and then return to starting position.

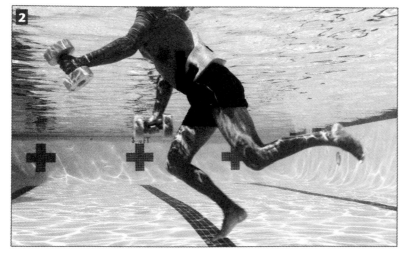

STARTING POSITION: With your feet off the bottom of the pool with or without a flotation device and with or without a tethered attachment, lean slightly forward. *Note:* An aqua belt can be worn around the midsection for support, or aqua bells can be placed under the armpits or held in each hand with the arms held to the side.

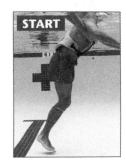

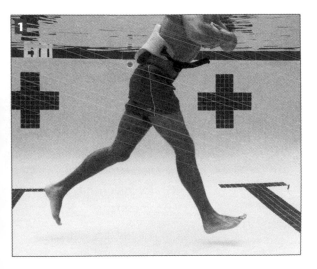

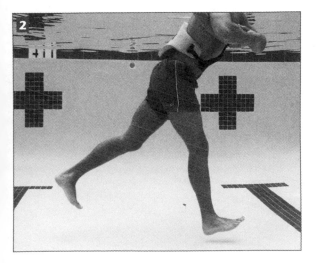

1–2 Keeping your legs fairly straight, slide them forward and backward as if cross-country skiing. The back leg should move back a comfortable distance—do not overstride.

You can also move your arms as follows:

- Pump your arms vigorously to obtain the intensity you desire.

- Punch both arms forward and really recoil them back.

- Act as if you're doing the crawl stroke but keep your arms underwater and pull your hand back as far as possible.

- Perform the breaststroke, pulling your arms hard.

- If you're untethered, use your arm motions to allow you to move a few feet forward and then return to starting position.

STARTING POSITION: With your feet off the bottom of the pool with or without a flotation device and with or without a tethered attachment, try to stay somewhat vertical.

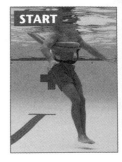

START

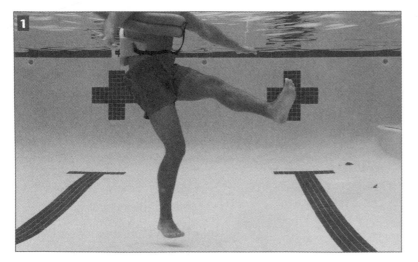

1–2 Keeping your legs straight, alternate swinging your legs forward as if you were a drum majorette. As you do so, move your arms as follows:

- Perform flies.

- Open your arms to the side then clap your hands to your chest (chest taps).

- Combine the flies with chest taps, alternating between the two.

- Combine breaststroke arms and hug arms.

- If you're untethered, use your arm motions to allow you to move a few feet forward and then return to starting position.

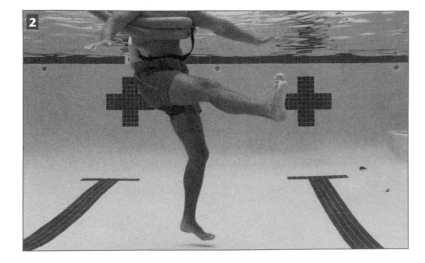

STARTING POSITION: With your feet off the bottom of the pool with or without a flotation device and with or without a tethered attachment, try to stay somewhat vertical.

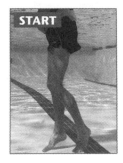

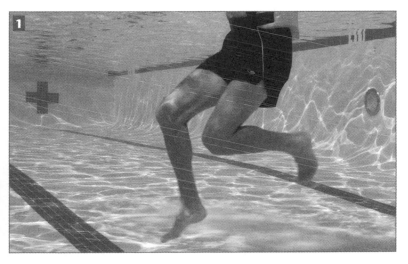

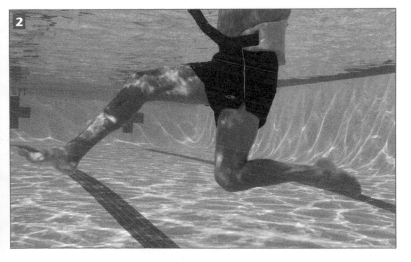

1–2 Move your legs as if you were kicking someone in front of you. As you do so, move your arms as follows:

- Punch your left arm forward as your left leg kicks, then alternate.

- Bring your right hand to your left knee.

- Move your arms as if you're doing the hula.

- Be creative and invent an arm motion that goes with the movement, your mood, or the music.

- If you're untethered, use your arm motions to allow you to move a few feet forward and then return to starting position.

deep-water sit-ups

target: midsection

These aren't as good as floor sit-ups but they're a lot more fun. Focus on using your abdominal muscles. Many people like to do this exercise with a noodle under their armpits.

STARTING POSITION: With your feet off the bottom of the pool either with or without a flotation device, lie on your back.

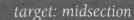

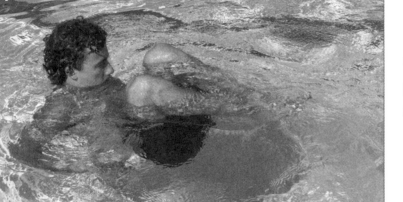

1 Bring your knees to your chest.

2 Extend your legs forward.

Repeat until you can't maintain proper form.

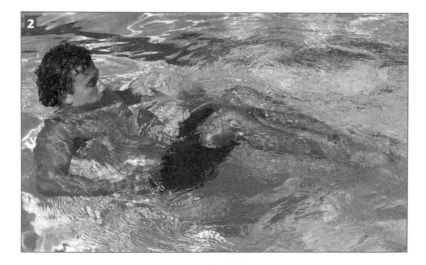

CAUTION: If you have lower back issues, be extra careful.

STARTING POSITION: With your feet off the bottom of the pool either with or without a flotation device, lie on your back.

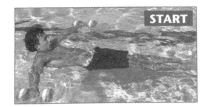

1 Bending your knees slightly, move your legs slightly to the left.

2 Return to center and move your legs slightly to the right.

Repeat until you can't maintain proper form.

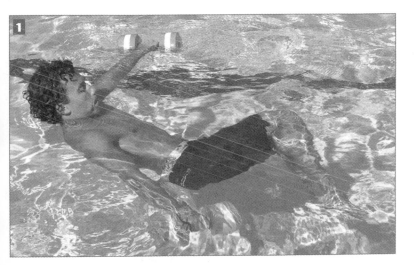

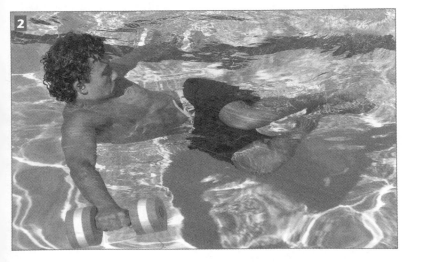

deep-water series

rock around the world

target: midsection, butt

CAUTION: If you have lower back issues, be extra careful.

STARTING POSITION: With your feet off the bottom of the pool either with or without a flotation device, lie on your back.

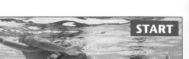

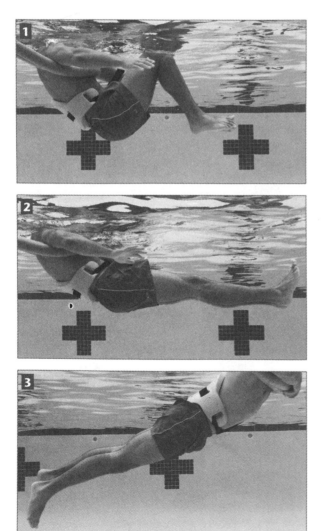

1 Bring your knees to your chest.

2 Extend your legs forward.

3 Pull your legs back in and extend them behind you.

hamstring stretch

THE STRETCH: Stand either with your back to the wall or unsupported in the water. Grasp one leg with both hands and pull your leg up. Straighten your leg, extend it forward and keep your toes pointed up. This stretch should be felt in the back of the thigh. Hold for 15–30 seconds.

Lower your leg back to starting position. Repeat with your other leg.

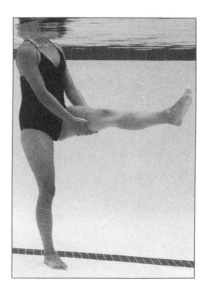

VARIATION: If you have trouble balancing, you can place your foot (toes up) on the wall.

calf stretch

target: calves

THE STRETCH: Place one hand on the wall for support. While keeping your heel down, slide your right leg straight back as far as possible. Bend your left knee slightly until the desired stretch is felt in your right calf muscle. Hold for 15–30 seconds.

Repeat on the other leg.

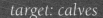

VARIATION: You can also do this by facing a wall and placing both hands on it for support.

stretches
ankle circles

STARTING POSITION: Stand either with your back to the wall or unsupported in the water.

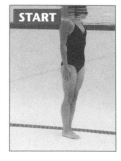

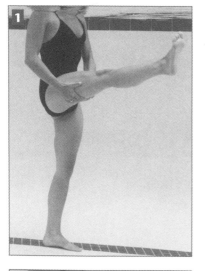

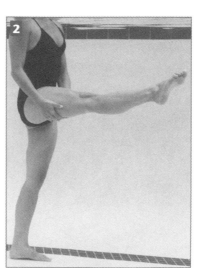

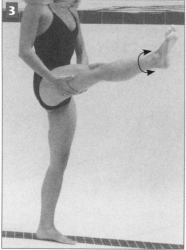

1 Grasp your right leg with both hands and pull your leg up. Keeping your leg straight, extend it forward and keep your toes pointed up. This stretch should be felt in the back of the thigh.

2 While keeping your leg stationary, point your foot forward and then pull it back several times. This motion will improve the range of motion of your ankle joint.

3 While keeping your leg stationary, draw circles in both directions with your foot.

Lower your leg back to starting position and repeat the sequence with your other leg.

STARTING POSITION: Stand tall with proper posture and place your right hand on your right shoulder and your left hand on your left shoulder.

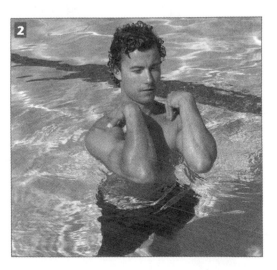

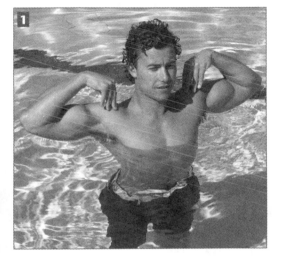

1 Keeping your hands in place, slowly take your elbows out to the sides as far as is comfortable. Hold for 5–15 seconds. Focus on squeezing your shoulder blades together and opening up your chest.

2 Bring your elbows together.

Repeat.

stretches
double wood chop

STARTING POSITION: Stand tall with proper neutral posture. Interlace your fingers in front of your body.

1 Inhale deeply through your nose while slowly lifting your arms as high as possible. Hold for 5–10 seconds.

Slowly lower your arms to starting position.

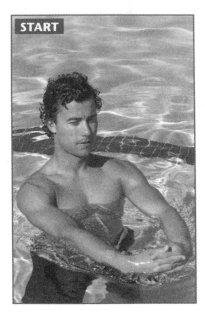

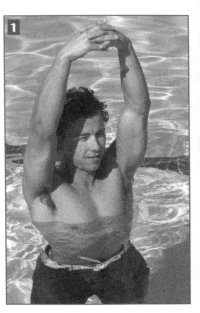

shoulder stretch

THE STRETCH: Stand tall with your feet comfortably apart. Take your right arm across your chest. Place your left hand just above your right elbow and gently press your elbow toward your throat. Hold for 5–10 seconds.

Repeat on the other side.

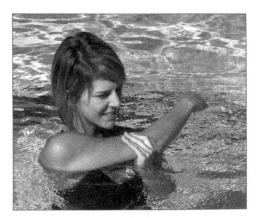

THE STRETCH: Stand tall with proper posture. Extend one arm in front of you at shoulder height, with your palm facing forward and fingers pointing up. With your other hand, gently pull your fingers back until the desired stretch is felt under your wrist. Hold for 10–15 seconds. Repeat on the other arm.

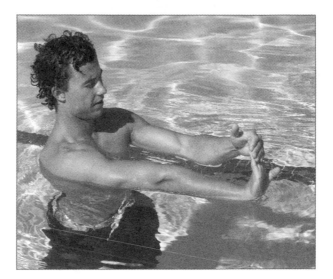

wrist stretch 2 *target: forearms*

THE STRETCH: Extend one arm in front of you at shoulder height, with your palm facing forward and fingers pointing down. With your other hand, gently pull your fingers back until the desired stretch is felt around your wrist. Hold for 10–15 seconds. Repeat on the other arm.

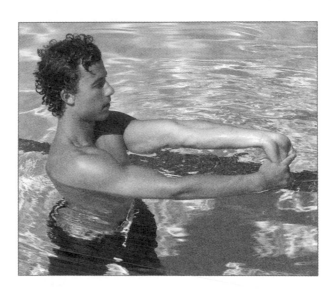

THE STRETCH: Stand with your back to the wall or unsupported in the water. Grasp one leg with both hands and bring your leg up to your chest. If it feels better, you can round your back. This movement should be felt in your lower back. Hold for 15–30 seconds.

Lower your leg to starting position and repeat with your other leg.

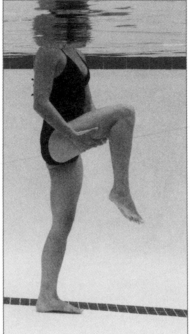

index

other ulysses press books

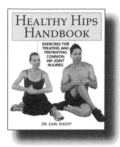

Healthy Hips Handbook
$14.95
Healthy Hips Handbook is designed to help prevent hip problems for some and, for those with existing hip problems, provide post-rehabilitation exercises.

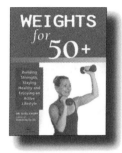

Weights for 50+
$14.95
Weight training is one of the most effective ways to get healthy and fight the physical signs of aging. *Weights for 50+* shows how easy it is for anyone to get started with weights.

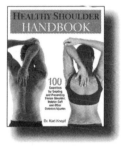

Healthy Shoulder Handbook
$15.95
Includes an overview of shoulder anatomy so anyone can use this friendly manual to strengthen an injured shoulder, identify the onset of a shoulder problem or better understand injury prevention.

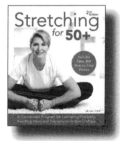

Stretching for 50+
2nd edition
$15.95
Details how readers can incorporate additional stretching to maintain flexibility, mobility and an active lifestyle.

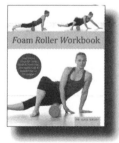

Foam Roller Workbook
$14.95
Details a comprehensive program for using the foam roller to recover from injury, reverse everyday pain and stay healthy in the future.

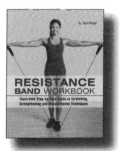

Resistance Band Workbook
$14.95
Amplify stretches and exercises for recovering from injury, increasing flexibility and building strength.

To order these books call 800-377-2542 or 510-601-8301, fax 510-601-8307, e-mail ulysses@ulyssespress.com, or write to Ulysses Press, PO Box 3440, Berkeley, CA 94703. All retail orders are shipped free of charge. California residents must include sales tax. Allow two to three weeks for delivery.

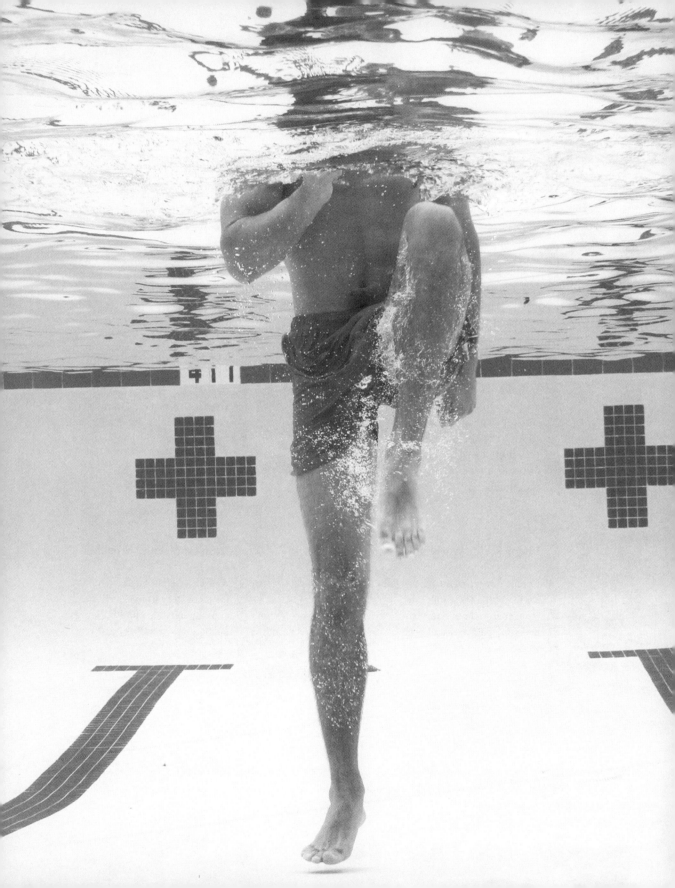

acknowledgments

This book would not have been possible without the expertise of Lily Chou and Claire Chun. Thanks to my models Sasha Wozniak, Kitty Chiu and Chris Knopf. Chris also provided insight into some of the water routines included in this book. A special thanks goes to Nancy Kao, executive director of the Forum at Rancho San Antonio, for allowing us the use of their magnificent facilities.

about the author

KARL KNOPF, author of *Foam Roller Workbook*, *Healthy Hips Handbook*, *Healthy Shoulder Handbook*, *Stretching for 50+*, *Weights for 50+* and *Total Sports Conditioning for Athletes 50+*, has been involved with the health and fitness of the disabled and older adults for 35 years. A consultant on numerous National Institutes of Health grants, Knopf has served as advisor to the PBS exercise series *Sit and Be Fit* and to the State of California on disabilities issues. He is a frequent speaker at conferences and has written several textbooks and articles. Knopf coordinates the Fitness Therapist Program at Foothill College in Los Altos Hills, California.